voices in my head

A Poetry Anthology

voices in my head - a poetry anthology

Copyright © 2024

All rights reserved.

Published by Red Penguin Books

Bellerose Village, New York

ISBN

Digital 978-1-63777-661-2

Print 978-1-63777-660-5

No part of this book may be reproduced in any form or by any electronic or mechanical means, including information storage and retrieval systems, without written permission from the author, except for the use of brief quotations in a book review.

contents

1. INSIDE YOUR HEAD — 1
Skye Ballantyne

2. COUNTING — 3
Kit Rose

3. THAT DAY. — 7
Shevaun Cavanaugh Kastl

4. VOICELESS — 11
Jessica Cook

5. AWAKENING — 13
Wanda W. Jerome

6. TUNED OUT — 15
Tinamarie Cox

7. STRENGTH IN TRAUMA — 17
Skye Ballantyne

8. CLIFFS OF SAGE — 19
Joshua Colenda

9. BE SUNSHINE — 23
Deepika Singh

10. JOY — 25
Michele Rule

11. BON VOYAGE — 27
Mary C. M. Phillips

12. MINOTAUR — 29
Dany Gagnon

13. BETWEEN WORLDS — 31
Cherie Hanson

14. LOST — 33
sally quon

15. LOST BUT NOT FOUND — 35
Skye Balentyne

16. MELISSA'S POEM — 37
Shai Afsai

17. HOW ARE YOU? Carol Edwards	39
18. PEARLS Joshua Colenda	43
19. EVENING PRAYER Jaki Sawyer	45
20. DARKNESS Michele Rule	47
21. HOW DO YOU EXPLAIN Skye Ballantyne	49
22. DARKNESS TO BE MADE LIGHT Mark Heathcote	51
23. SUFFOCATING Skye Ballantyne	53
24. THE MAELSTROM Janet Rudolph	55
25. WISHINGS Carol Edwards	57
26. PENMANSHIP Joshua Colenda	61
27. PILLOW Matt Mcgee	63
28. HEARTACHE Wanda W. Jerome	65
29. LET ME LET GO Skye Ballantyne	67
30. ENTRY 7: DEPRESSION DIARY Lisa Diaz Meyer	69
31. DAMAGED Natasha Alva	71
32. SNOW Sally Quon	73
33. AM I THE ONE WHO SAYS I AM Michele Rule	75
34. LOCKSMITH Dany Gagnon	77

35. THE STEWING Joshua Colenda	79
36. BIGGEST FEAR Skye Ballantyne	81
37. SOUL THERAPY Lanzz Linked	83
38. WHEN YOUR EYES ARE INFRARED Mark Heathcote	85
39. CHEERLESS MORNING Michele Rule	87
40. EVER-PRESENT (AFTER VAN MORISON) Jacob Moses	89
41. IRREPARABLE Carol Edwards	91
42. BOB Matt Mcgee	93
43. HATE YOU Skye Ballantyne	95
44. SELF-HELP LETTER FROM A FRIEND Self-Help Letter from a Friend	97
45. WORDS Sally Quon	99
46. WHERE I'M CALLING FROM Eran F. S. D. Hornick	101
47. THE TASTE OF YOU Dany Gagon	105
48. WAKING NIGHTMARE Skye Ballantyne	107
49. BEDTIME STORIES Tinamarie Cox	109
50. GREY MOTH Mark Heathcote	111
51. LEARNED TO ENJOY MYSELF Henry Vinicio Valerio Madriz	113
52. THE ISLAND Joshua Colenda	115

53. HAPPINESS WILL FIND YOU   117
Skye Ballantyne

54. ASYLUM   119
Olivia Arieti

55. UMBRELLAS   121
Michele Rule

56. BRIGHTEST SHADE OF GREY   123
Sally Quon

57. MICE ARE SENSITIVE   125
Carol Edwards

58. THE BORDER OF US   127
Michael Artemis

59. SEASONAL AFFECTIVE DISORDER (SAD)   129
Mark Heathcote

60. HEARTBREAKER   131
Joshua Colenda

61. PEACE   133
Skye Ballantyne

62. TO THE POPULAR SOUL WHO FEELS UNLOVED   135
Michelle Chermaine Ramos

63. 10:30   137
Natasha Alva

64. ADDICTION DIARY: ENTRY 4: DETOX   139
Lisa Diaz Meyer

65. IMPULSE   141
Michael Artemis

66. VILLAIN INSIDE   143
Skye Ballantyne

67. LOVE IS A BATTLEFIELD: A DIALOGUE   145
William John Rostron

68. STATIC   149
Michelle Chermaine Ramos

69. UNTIL YOU'VE SUFFERED WITH IT   151
Mark Heathcote

70. DISORDER   153
Olivia Arieti

71. FIREWORKS — 155
Michele Rule

72. THE DAY AFTER — 157
Michael Artemis

73. DEMIGOD — 161
Joshua Colenda

74. COMFORTING YOU — 165
Skye Ballantyne

75. UNENDING — 167
Carol Edwards

76. THE HUNDRED YEAR WAR — 169
Shevaun Cavanaugh Kastl

77. SÉANCE — 173
Alex Grehy

78. BECAUSE I AM A LIAR — 175
Carol Edwards

79. ARE YOU ALIVE? — 177
Skye Ballantyne

80. DEAR OLD DEAD JULY — 179
Mark Heathcote

81. TIGHTROPE — 181
Alex Grehy

82. INTERNAL MONOLOGUE — 183
Carol Edwards

83. SELF-DESTRUCTION — 185
Skye Ballantyne

84. HIDE — 187
Carol Edwards

85. KIND EYES AND THE LOVELIEST FACE I'D EVER SEEN — 189
Gabriella Balcom

86. FEEL ALIVE — 191
Skye Ballentyne

87. IT'S NOT ME WHO WROTE THIS, — 193
Aditya Pandey

88. BROKEN GLASS — 195
Carol Edwards

89. KILLING THE MINOTAUR Dany Gagnon	197
90. SCARED TO HEAL Skye Ballantyne	199
About the Authors	201
Also from The Red Penguin Collection	209

Inside Your Head

- Skye Ballantyne

Depression is silent,
It creeps up on you,
Slowly,
Little by little.
You never hear it,
You never see it.
Until suddenly,
It's the loudest voice
Inside your head.

It's screaming
At the top of its lungs.
Refusing,
To be ignored.
Sometimes,
The worst place,
You can be,
Is in
Your own head.

Counting

By Kit Rose

They matched on a Wednesday; a Wednesday evening specifically. Sam remembered that it was a Wednesday because her anxiety forced her to keep diligent records of the passing days while he remained in her life. Another Wednesday meant another threshold crossed, and the worry of him joining the ranks of her ghosts surged and subsided all at once. The fear of allowing herself to feel clawed at her chest, ripping away hope as it would flutter by. Afterall, how meaningful of a connection could one make on Bumble?

By the first Friday, they had moved over to Snapchat. His responses were scattered throughout the next week, always coupled with an apology and the insistence that he'd been busy. Logically, she understood and assured herself there was no reason not to believe him. The inner demons whispered otherwise. Drawing herself into a hug with her knees pressed to her chest, Sam whispered to herself, "if he didn't want to talk, he wouldn't respond at all." But, her long list of heartbreaks dug themselves out of their graves and taunted her with reminders of how quickly things can fall apart. The universe had cursed her, dangling happy endings to grace her fingertips and yanking it away so her hands bled. With a sniff, she curled into her pillow and blew away the mental tornado.

With the arrival of the second Saturday came the transition to texting. Sam was satisfied with the upgrade, soothing herself with the slight permanence this had. The lump in her throat shrank, almost small enough to swallow. The demons lay in wait, peeking out of her subconscious. Their hissed chants carried themselves to the forefront of her mind, allowing a dark cloud to loom over her comfort.

. . .

"It'll end. It'll end. It'll end."

She shook her head in defiance as the three dots signified he was typing.

"It'll end. It'll end. It'll end."

She deflated as the dots disappeared.

On the second Tuesday, the two spent the day playing rounds of virtual cup pong and 8-ball up until after midnight. He bid Sam goodnight with a cheerful, "thanks for game night; I thoroughly enjoyed it." A brief smile slipped through Sam's composure before a wave of anger washed it away. *Stop. No. It's too new.* It had only been two Tuesdays. That was nowhere near long enough to smile. That was nowhere near long enough to feel anything.

Midnight struck on the third Sunday and the whirlwind of distress pillaged through Sam's veins. They still had not met, they still had not FaceTimed, there was no chance this wasn't going to end in tears. Her worry of being in too deep had morphed into an all consuming monster. The storm leaked from her eyes and gripped her throat as she hovered her finger over the 'block' button. She could end this right now. Rip off the bandaid. Escape before truly investing. That was the smart thing to do. That was the way that Sam could protect herself, and it was her obligation to protect herself. She could escape the ticking clock beating in her chest; the endless wondering if they'd make it to another Wednesday. It *ticked* and *ticked* and *ticked*. Turning off her phone, she buried her face in her sheets until the sun rose.

The fourth Wednesday greeted her like the checkpoint of a marathon, fully stocked with water and sweat rags. The monster roared and spat fire as she bit her lip in the face of the mirror. Wednesday number five brought along 'good morning' and 'goodnight', paired with smiley faces or hearts. For every smile, the monster grew larger, following Sam tirelessly with its bellowing huffs. The monster sat between them at the movies on the seventh Friday. It lived under the restaurant table on the ninth Saturday. On the tenth Thursday, it taunted the lack of a label on their relationship as Sam tried desperately to sleep.

But, then Sam lost count.

On a Wednesday, a Wednesday evening specifically, they stood on the doorstep of his childhood home where she would meet his parents for the first time. Turning to face her, he prepared himself to knock. "Are you ready?" A pang of nerves struck her, holding her tongue. He squeezed Sam's hand, looking into her eyes with a reassuring grin. "They're going to love you." Letting out a cleansing breath, she gave him a nod. As he knocked on the door, Sam stole a glance behind her.

The monster wasn't there.

That day.

- Shevaun Cavanaugh Kastl

February
    A Wednesday
        In a year I can't recall...

It was so hard to move that day.
The crushing weight of shame and fear. Galvanized, dread made steel.
Surrounded by phantoms,
Counting heartbeats as heartstrings danced to the grave
    Melody of a Victorian funeral dirge.

But while my body fell heavy,
My conscience was conscious.
Moral banister engaged and alert And Manic with self-recrimination.
    I was sick to death of me.

Selfish, self possessed
Or obsessed... I can't discern
The difference as clearly as I used to.
It began as a pinprick in my chest, And a slow bleed of molten fire
Before paralyzing every nerve, every muscle of propulsion,
In still life poses like the stone ruins of Oz.

But Dorothy returned home, didn't she? Ruby slippers, three careless clicks, And one wishful entreaty.

    There's no place like home,
    There's no place like home...

But I can't remember how to get there. Switching tenses in time,
Now my feet are bare and too tired to click So my heels never part from the ground.

I want to pray,
    But then I must breathe,
        And I don't want to feel *that* pain. That crushing intake of air that rips at the seam of the armor guarding my heart Like a chink in chainmail and a slow, painful
death.
But one cannot live without breath,
    And I have always wanted to Live. So I close my eyes and squeeze.

And I'm seven and clutching my mother's hand
As a needle pricks my arm.
Do I know that I'm
Doomed to chronic remembrance of past lives and messes,
Steadfast regressing- Always forgetting the present moment
 When I'm
 In.
Doomed to slowly spectate
As it all falls away
Like grains of sand through a sieve.
    Will I remember this?

I'm guessing I won't since I can feel the nylon (fabric) pull.

So I reach and I twist
Orange plastic, white cap.
One, not enough,
    Two is too much.
        So three should manage nicely.
I know better, of course.
It's the thing that haunts me,
But I Need a second
To not think,
    To not feel,
        To not know-
And so,

Hand moves to mouth and I swallow, Slowly relenting my grip on reality Before blissful oblivion and a skip in time.

Going,
   Going,
      Gone.

Voiceless

- Jessica Cook

"I don't hear voices," I say to the psychiatrist
And he takes that to mean I am not mentally ill
Unfortunately I do think that they're going to burn me as a witch
I think that I can tell the future and something catastrophically bad
Is going to happen to me and everyone I know.
But I don't say any of that.
I think that Extinction Rebellion are out to get me.
Or maybe it's a cult
Perhaps I am on a TV show of my life
Everyone is tracking me at all times.
A Truman Show.
Maybe if I walk far enough I will reach the edge of the dome.
I think that the telly is communicating
Messages just for me.
Spotify is sending me clues
About the web of conspiracies around me.
I think that the whole internet has
Been written to mock me.
I think that
The hospital is a cult
And I've been kidnapped
But I tell him over and over
That the only voice I hear
Is my internal monologue
Quiet and not really a voice at all
Just my thoughts
banging around in there.
Endlessly.

AWAKENING
by
Wanda W. Jerome

ABUNDANCE   NOTHING NEEDED   PEACEFUL MOMENT
PERFECT
DEEP   BLISS   WATER   FLOWING
CRYSTAL BLUE SKY   CLOUDS STREAMING
SO PRECIOUS   SO LOVELY   SO PROFOUND
IN THIS PLACE   OUTSIDE IS IN AND THROUGH
LIFE INHALES EACH AND ALL   WE RESPOND IN KIND
JOY RADIATES   BLESSINGS ABOUND
THE PATH   CIRCULAR   SPIRALING OUT AND IN
SEE   TASTE   TOUCH   FEEL   HEAR
BUBBLING   GURGLING   LIVING   BREATHING
ECSTACY IN MOTION
PUT ASIDE THE DOING FOR NOW
NOW IS EVERYTHING   EVER WAS AND WILL BE
SILKEN BALM FOR THE HUMAN SOUL
STAND IF YOU CAN
REACH   GIVE   FEEL   SMILE
BEAMING BE
WHAT JOY   WHAT BLISS
WE ARE BEAUTIFUL
WE ARE ONE
LIVE LIFE IN COLORS OF AWARENESS
LIMITLESS   BOUNDLESS
FREE FROM FOGGY DREAMS OF SEPARATENESS AND PAIN
BEING WAITS FOR US IN MOMENTS SO LIGHT
WE RISE UP – UP
DARING TO REACH   BEYOND THE STARS
SHIMMERING   GOLDEN
FROTHY BUBBLES RIDING THE WAVES
WE DANCE ON THE OCEAN OF THE UNIVERSE

Tuned Out

- Tinamarie Cox

Why aren't you listening to how loud I'm screaming?
The sound thrashing and crashing against the walls.
Like I want to do with my fragile body.
Shattering the windows with my voice.
Spraying the notes and glass down into your eardrums.
It's me, all alone in my bedroom, again.
Emanating a deafening silence.
With music pulsing into my ears, coursing through my veins.
After giving up on anybody hearing me.
Slowly fading out with the last song.

Strength In Trauma

By Skye Ballantyne

They say my trauma made me stronger, it gave me strength and built me into what I am. No! I want to shout and tell the world. My trauma made me traumatized. It made me weak. It made me break down at the simplest things. It stole my sleep and happy memories. It made me tremble and shake and feel things I never wanted to feel. It made me remember things I never even wanted to experience in the first place. My trauma didn't give me strength. My trauma broke me. It made me a shell of my former self.

I made myself strong. I was the person who made me who I am, by picking up the broken pieces and pulling myself out of the darkness as I pieced together the pieces that someone else had caused.

Cliffs of Sage

By: Joshua Colenda

I open my eyes to see the world,
Broken in my mirror.
My heart yearns for a better one.

The path is steep,
And soon I find myself beset by bandits,
Ruining my plans,
They cast me into despair.

This time I open my eyes to darkness.
I am cushioned by a bed of corpses:
The others who have tried.
I started this journey to fix what I could see,
But if I lay here,
With the others who have failed,
Soon, the world will not bother me.

An ancient rumble rouses me from sleep,
It asks if I have finished failing.
It says if I am humble,
It will teach me all it knows,
And feed me what it grows.
But if I become arrogant,
Or burdened by my foolishness,
I will fall into an even deeper pit than this.

'Teach me, train me, beat me, lead me!',
I called out to the sage.
I told him I was not afraid,
But he did not believe me.

Six years passed in that ravine,
Where every day I tried to be,
The good the sage said he saw in me.

Six years passed before I could say goodbye,
Before I was free to live,
And he,
To die.

He crept into a hole,
A grave,
And I,
Alone but for his gifts,
Turned my gaze once more upon the cliffs.

With my new vision I could see,
The cliffs were not as solid as they seemed.
And with the wisdom of the sage,
I began to chip away.

But still it was not easy.
The winds whipped from all around,
To knock me from the cliffs,
And onto the ground.

Wildlife came to test me.
Scavengers would bite me if I dropped my guard,
And predators would kill me.

For twenty-eight days I climbed that rock,
Making little progress,
Carving uncomfortable beds out of stone.

Finally,
I stood upon the summit,
And I could see it all!
Below me was the pit,
With all of those the cliffs had broken,
And the teacher who had helped me live.

On my right I saw a river,
Which wound its way to the horizon.

But so much illumination,
Sent me to my knees,
I had to close my eyes,
To keep it all from blinding me.

And as I sat there,
In the darkness of my thoughts,
At the peak of my success,
I heard every wind that ever tried to knock me off my path,
Together ask,
'But where will you sleep tonight?'

Be Sunshine

- Deepika Singh

My buzzing mind is plagued by anxiety.
Sometimes it's more than I can handle
And it makes me feel numb
It follows me like a shadow, a curse.
I am so lost in the meandering world
Heart pumps out, voice choked down.
My lips tremble to utter a word
As you may advertise my long unending trauma
A smallest alter in your tone, my feet tremble
And I end up in full of fright
Deep down my heart always begging for some light
We dwell in our mental health
So don't make it a wretched hell
Don't expect others to heal your wound
Rise like a Tiger and roar like a Lion
Sparkle yourself and get a brand new yourself.

Joy

- Michele Rule

When all I feel is darkness
thick greasiness
   ungraspable
all scent   taste
sound dulled down
   memory drowning
pulled down
an ocean of despair
some images life jacket me
all the sky colours
cloud, sun, moon
greys   blues   azures
night, day, dusk
all the growth shades
 a spring-tail in the March snow
a husky puppy
bouncing like that
any new fragile life
the first time I held my granddaughter

Bon Voyage

I will take along a spirit of adventure
and leave my fear behind

I will pack healthy thoughts
and place all second guessing

in an old battered suitcase
the one with the wonky zipper

never to be opened
or frustrated upon again

I will carry the belief that
I have simply done my best

and leave the nettling regrets
at the baggage claim

destined to circle
round and round and round

but, without me

- Mary C. M. Phillips

Minotaur

- Dany Gagnon

Minotaur
Ariadne where is your golden thread
that I may stitch my life
and fall asleep
without dreaming of monsters

Between Worlds
- Cherie Hanson

My heart walks the desert
upside down dizzy with stars under foot.
They are not sharp piercing my flesh.
I feel their cold blue flatness receiving me.
I am lost in the wilderness between two great expanses.
"Why have you forsaken me," I cry out to the emptiness.

Reality is segmented with no vanishing point
no two silver steel rails touching
at one point to show the ceasing to exist.

I calm myself with questions
wrapping my arms around myself to define the measurement of now.

It is worse than chaos, this loosening of the old structures of story.

In the past, I lay in a crib abandoned to the hospital.
The white nurses moved to me like polar bears.
I was caged forever alone without a beating pulse.

The uniformity of nothingness:
My father driving the eternity of desert at night.
I remember,
when I was 14,
sitting backseat hypnotized by the vacuum of not one sighted structure
to anchor me,
hour after hour.

The slide down the birth canal to the stinging sand
head down endurance
attempting survival
from the first un-recollected moments.

Yesterday, my friend said, "Your life is not a concentration camp."

lost

- sally quon

lost
in pieces
of shattered glass
reflection distorted
memory curves
and distills
edges coloured by time
there is nothing here
reminiscent
of what was real
only a fading memory
it was ever here at all
self-defense
cratering within the
brain lobes
synapses sparking
the lingering light
flashes behind my eyes

Lost But Not Found

By Skye Ballantyne

It doesn't feel real.
I don't feel real.
I'm sitting there, watching.

People are talking around me.
No one knows.
We haven't told them.

Life goes on.
Plans move forward.
It's as if everything is going to stay the same, but it's not.

Things are changing
Far too quickly.
Things are changing
and I'm suffocating.

They just go on
as if my world wasn't crumbling. Nothing's real.

Nothing matters.
Nothing really exists.
I'm just this shell.

This empty thing
drifting, endlessly drifting.
In and out of consciousness.

In and out.
Lost but not found

Melissa's Poem

By Shai Afsai

Mom is scheduled to call
in about an hour.
I open a bottle of wine.

———

On the second date,
I express an opinion.
It's over.

———

I meet up with three friends for cocktails,
just like the girls from *Sex and the City* —
except we're not in New York, and I don't like my friends.

———

Making the bed alone,
the sheets won't stay in place.
But he never helped with that either.

———

Clearly the woman on the mat to my right
is convinced deodorant and yoga
are mutually exclusive.

———

He explains that women keep living longer
and men are dying younger.
I sleep with him anyway.

———

Now I have a thing for guys with beards —
but after a few weeks or a month, I push them to shave.
They do, and we break up soon after.

———

Driving back from my sister's,
I remember:
I hated her even when we were kids.

———

He's muscled, with arms covered in tattoos,

and tells me that the more he looks like an ex-con,
the more women are drawn to him. I'm drawn.

———

He tells me he divorced his second wife after she allowed
his stepdaughter to buy a pet rabbit over his objections.
Somehow this makes sense to me.

———

He says he spent three months in the far east,
and that yoga changed his life.
I trick myself into believing I've met someone interesting.

———

He's twelve years older. Before #MeToo, I'd have told women
he was my former high school teacher, just to get a reaction,
and half of them would've said, "That's hot!"

———

Xanax inside
the white pharmacy bag —
no need to die now.

How are you?

by Carol Edwards

                                                    "How are you," they ask
                                                                 Tired, I say

So tired
Exhausted
Bone tired
    Not sleepy; I'm awake, I'm working, functioning
    But the heaviness in my chest
    The lump in my throat that threatens
    To come out as tears
        As screams
        As sighs
                Sighs of resignation, of surrender, of sadness
    The fuzziness behind my eyes
    The cords tightening in my neck
    Strain my head, my brain, my thoughts
        My words
            My   hope...

Burdens stoop my shoulders
    Ruin my posture
    Ergonomic nightmare
Burdens
    Burden of responsibility
    Of reliability
    Of breadwinning
        Winning but somehow
        Always losing
Burden of perfection, flawless expectation
Burden of loving, wanting love
        Feeling too much
                Wishing I could feel little
                      Yet knowing that changes who I am...

Who am I?
      Why am I here?
            What am I doing these things for?
This weight sits and settles on me
Day after day
Hour after hour
      Minutes seem hours
           Excruciating lifetimes
Feeling
      Everything
    Yet nothing matters
      (Or so the sadness tells me...)

Sometimes I only find relief in tears
    Not even in sleep
        In sleep, my thoughts don't have me
        To stop them
            Dreamless isn't a thing I do
            Dream full, always
                Just whether I remember when
I wake up
Tired, so tired
Bone tired, I don't say

                                    Just tired, I say
                                    Busy, I say

Busy to keep the thoughts away
    Busy to feel less

                                          Busy

Working, talking, helping, walking
      Voraciously reading
            Crying
        Alone...

                              "How are you," they ask

                                                    Tired, I say

And walk away
They don't actually want to know
            (The sadness claims)
Burden of perfection
        Burden of strength and survival
                Burdens I should never have had to bear
                                        Alone.
I just want to rest
                (I'll rest when I'm dead.)
                                        (Will I?)
Sometimes Death appears
The deepest rest enough
But it says I can't yet,
        "I know you're tired
        But not yet."

Original version first published in Shards (The Ravens Quoth Press, 2024)

Pearls
By: Joshua Colenda

What hope have we,
The hopeless,
That is not already,
In our souls?

I am like an oyster,
Cold,
And shut,
And grey.
But inside,
Pink,
And lively!
Turning the irritants of consciousness,
Into something great.

So give me all the trials of this world,
And I will give you pearls.

Evening Prayer

by Jaki Sawyer

Now that sleep is no longer frightening,
no looming nightmare,
dark formless terrors,
I can admire, even love
slow sinking of the sun,
deepening dark that follows.
Moon, stars, the sound of water,
wind in branches,
sleepy robin,
song sparrow that sings til dawn.

Those things I did
that are not evil,
but bad, yes, from ignorance or sloth,
lazy will, stupid giving in -
those things that I regret but
must acknowledge -
I have paid with many sleepless nights.
Let it go then, accepted
to fade into falling night.
Let evening spread as comfort.
Let me forgive myself.

Darkness

Night comes down like a sledgehammer
and the stars hide.
Everything is crushed by thunder,
pounding rain and shrieks of wind.
The house creaks, windows rattle,
blackness haphazardly ripped by demon flashes
from the horror of my past.
I think there was summer once and
if there was, then sunshine, birdsong, leaf rustle -
perhaps a cardinal calling 'pretty, pretty'
before flitting to the feeder and a blue jay
scolding down-
if that place still exists, or ever did,
where red-breasted nuthatch peeks
upside down at the brown creeper,
where the hardest thing you have to do
is fill that feeder and shoo
away the squirrels –
    where was that?
Was it a real place?

How Do You Explain

By Skye Ballantyne

It's easier to stay quiet.
It's easier to not say a word.
After all, how could you explain,
When you didn't even understand it yourself?

How did you explain
How you were both happy and sad?
You were lost and confused
And yet calm and content?

How did you explain
That you felt everything
And yet nothing at all?
You can't.

It's easier to stay quiet.
It's easier to just laugh,
To smile,
To act like everything is fine.

But it's all a lie.
Behind that smile,
Behind the laughter,
Behind the quiet,
Was a broken heart,
Were tears,
Were emotions raging so loudly
They drowned out everything else.

How do you explain,
How you don't feel good enough
For anyone
Not even yourself?

How do you explain
Why you would forgive over and over again
Someone who never truly saw your worth,
Simply because you felt you deserved it -
Because you didn't see your own worth?

How do you explain,
That you broke your own heart?
By believing in false promises
By someone who would never truly value you?

How do you explain,
That all you want to do,
Is to stop feeling?
Because not feeling would be better
Than the constant pain
Of a self-inflicted heart break.

How do you explain
When you don't understand it yourself?

Darkness to be made light

by Mark Heathcote

Without hell, there's no heaven.
Yes, there is a darkness to be made light again
Anyone who has not suffered from low self-esteem
or depression, all know it's an endless fight back
to good health; black clouds flock like vultures
for the bread of our souls
and the flesh of our hearts
to peck out the seed of our visionary eyes.
But we wheeled an axe of our reasoning
an axe of own fortitude
it's our own minds' insight that threads the pieces
back together like a steel cable car bridge
reaching across the dark expanse of despair
this is when we begin to know ourselves again
all our hopes-fulfillment and who we are?

Suffocating

By Skye Ballantyne

I'm suffocating.
I can't breathe.
Pain is pulling me under.
Drowning me.

I'm coughing up water,
I'm drowning,
Begging for your help,
Begging for my life.

I'm drowning,
And you're standing
Three feet away,
Screaming, "learn how to swim."

I'm suffocating,
I'm drowning,
I'm dying,
And you don't care.

THE MAELSTROM

by Janet Rudolph

I walk outside into a blustery windstorm.
My clothing whips about me as my unbound hair flies into an agitated, wild tangle.

This turbulent maelstrom gains steam.
I am in my element.
My visceral fury mirrors the rhythm of this encircling ferocity.
My stinging skin pores form the connecting bridge between my insides and the disintegrating vista, fueling each other to greater and greater heights.

I cheer the encompassing chaos, "Go wild, go free."
Even as my shouted words dissolve into the howling gale.

Stepping out further into the street to feel its gathering force unimpeded,
I enjoy the tortured movement of the trees writhing as if to escape such madness.

A loose shutter from somewhere bangs into my consciousness adding rough harmony to the clamor.
Oh! the joy of being in the nucleus of this potent destruction!

But then, without warning my young son is standing at my side.
In horror, I wonder, how he got out here?
Should I prevent his tender eyes from viewing such ruinous force?
He looks at me with curious intent, observing all this horror and ugliness. I cannot move for a timeless brief moment.

"Oh mommy," he cries, his tiny innocent face seeking mine.

Have my anger and the wind already pierced him? Is it too late to shield him?

How could this have happened?

I hear him yelling above the noise, "Look, mommy," his chubby finger pointing, his eyes shining with excitement, "The trees, they're dancing!"

Wishings

by Carol Edwards

"I wish
    I wish"
I wish to change something
    Change something about this life
        This God-given life
            This tainted-by-my-choices life
      That is un-satisfactory
      That is un-fortunately
        Un-acceptable
      To my current sensibilities.

I wish
    I wish
On stars, on burning meteorites
On fluffy dandelions
On necklace clasps touching pendants
On found pennies
    Picked up, maybe flipped up
    Arcing
        Into some fountain
    The shine winking at the universe
      All secret-like
      Coy thing
      Bribing Fate to come for a visit
      "A little something for your time
        Pay me no mind."

I wish
    I wish
On triple digits, or quadruple
    Twice a day
"Make" this or that "go away"
    "Come back"

> "Happen"
>> "End in my favor"

All these wishings a form of prayer
To a god we have no use for
But treat as Luck or Chance or however
You want to call it, just not God
    Who gives Life.

I wish
    I wish
I could redo my life
What I hold in my hands today
Is a broken music box that used to play
    A doll that used to dance
    A heart that used to beat, beat, beat
        Until fear took its drum, and anger its bass
            A desperate searching-longing-what-is-my
                Meaning
    Took its timing
    Its sight, hearing
So blind and dumb it stumbles toward this thrum-
    -ing violin string
        Singing
"I wish
    I wish."

I wish for the life she has, he has
    For the words, prophesies, eloquence
    Pieces of creative dust somehow
    Denied me
I wish for lands, sands
    The security of fences
        (This is mine, you cannot have)
    Of sense and cents
        (wisdom and all those pennies
            In a piggy bank the size of a mountain)
I wish for the stars (and starts) and the moon and sun
    To come at the smallest beckon

   Of my hand
I wish to knit souls and cells
   And break them, too
I wish for the grand crescendo
    The final fight where I overcome
     The villain, the threat, the Evil
      Alone
    Proving self-sufficient power, purpose   peace.

I wish
  I wish
Then,   sometimes,   for no wishes at all
Just the quiet unmaking
Of my birth,   my death
My existence,   that I'd have never
Left the brand, the burn, the cut of me
On Time and Life
      Un-worthy.

Penmanship
By: Joshua Colenda

My pen,
My truest friend,
Turns the world into a message,
Only I can send.
Into a shape,
That only I can bend.
Into a wound,
That only I can mend.

And to my page I say,
"Let the truth sink in.
Like a slow tattoo,
You've always had me,
And I'll always have you."

PILLOW

By Matt Mcgee

The night after Mac died,
a text dinged in my cell phone.
"I think I'm losing it," Shelley said.
"I'm alone. My roomie's at his girlfriend's
and I have nowhere to go." From the
curb outside her house,
I dialed her cell:

"Hello?"
"Come unlock the door."
"OK."

She led the way to her bedroom.
"Now don't be weird about this,"
and I suspected we were about to cover
the male-female mourning ground rules,
but she grabbed a pillow off her bed;
it wore one of Mac's dirty t-shirts.
She shoved it under my nose.

"Look, it smells like him.
I've been lying here, napping with it.
I slept on his bed last night."

I kicked off my shoes, fell onto her bed
and she burrowed into my chest. "We're just
going to lie here," I said, "all three of us."
She laughed and snugged in, Mac's dressed-up
pillow pulled against her. She babbled, cried,
mourned. Most of what she said didn't
require wisdom, or even an answer,
just an ear to hear it unravel.

HEARTACHE
by
Wanda W. Jerome

ROUND   SAD-FACED SHADE   OBSCURE   SLANTED EYES
TALL   SHORT   BROKEN   SPRAWLING GREEN   LEGS
ARMS   ARROWS   ROOTS   VEINS
LIVING   BLOOD-CRUSTED   FEATHERED LEAVES
BROWN   GOLDEN   CRUMBLED   SWEPT UP
WINDLACED SUMMER NIGHTS

BRIGHT LIGHT   FLAWED FAWN   FROWNING
FORGIVING YELLOW HUES   TILTED   BRUISED
ALL KNOWING   ALL SEEING   ALL BEINGS BLUE
REFLECTED IN NARROW PECULIAR SHADOWS
TREASURES NEVER FOUND
INSIDE-UP AND DOWN
HILLSIDE MASSACRE IN MOONLIGHT

WILDLIFE PLAYS   WATER DROPS BEIGE
HEARTSTRINGS FALL APART IN A RAGE
WINTERING   SUMMER FROZEN IN TIME
MEMORIES OF PURE SPRINGS
MEANDERING THROUGH BRUISED CHEEKS
BROKEN SURFACE   SILKEN SOFT LIGHT
FIRE FACE
REFLECTING THE TRAIL OF TEARS

CRAGS OF CRACKS OUTSTRETCHED
GREEN-WHITE MOSSES CLING
A HUMAN KNIFE MOVES SWIFTLY IN THE GLOW OF THE
GLOBE
THESE TREES FEEL   MIDNIGHT
THEY BEND AND RISE
HOLDING FORCED HUMAN HEARTS   CARVED TO
STAND OUT

WATERS POUR FROM THE HUMAN EYE RIVER
CATCH A GLIMPSE OF THE GLOBE IN THE TREES
SHAPE CUT WITH DAGGER-LIKE PRECISION IN THE
NIGHT
MOUNTAINS IN LOVERS' EYES
ROUND   PROBING   DISTANCING   CUTTING
A KNIFE IN THE HEART OF THE NIGHT
LIKE MOON IN TREES

Let Me Let Go

By Skye Ballantyne

My world is caving
Breaking me down.

Where do you run,
When you're at your limit?

So tired of feeling,
I'm letting you down.

Now I feel guilty,
For running out of time.

Running through Hell,
Looking for an escape.

So tired of trying,
Let me let go.

Entry 7: Depression Diary

By Lisa Diaz Meyer

Whose thoughts
Have crept into my head...
The writing vessel leaks its dark ink
Staining the lined
And feathered crevices
Of my hand
Rocking motions
Are meant to soothe
Close my eyes
I cannot look
I once wore the face of sanity

Damaged

by: Natasha Alva

Broken windows, scattered papers, shredded sheets,
tilted paintings, dusty shelves, and wrecked furniture.
I don't care, I'm in a maze that I can't escape.
I'm a mess, please do not mind my pain.
Baggy eyes, purple bruises, bloody knife wounds and fiery burns.
Strangely, there's no more pain.
I don't feel anything.
Always the target, being hit around and played,
There're no such things as kindness in this world.
Why am I still breathing?
Undermined and insulted until I'm buried to the ground,
now there's no confidence, so why question that as if you're the victim.
Being called a bad influence, treated as an outcast.
A face of all the gossip, becoming a wretched mess until they see your tears.
I tried standing still too long, but I'm tired of fighting.
Nobody listens, talks, or even remembers me.
What's the use of my being if I'm just damaged goods?
Please get me out of this prison, I'm ready to go.
I'm damaged, damaged, damaged.
I'm just a ragged little doll with no life anymore.
It's hard to hold it in when you're labelled as a stranger.
With no guidance and help, I'm a lost stray.
Sitting in a corner with just these ugly scars, waiting for tears to pour out but nothing comes out.
I tried to stick to the rules, but not everything went to plan.
I might need to not wake up in case it all goes sideways.
Tired of holding all the fake smiles, pretending nothing happens.
Please get me out of this prison, I'm ready to go.

Snow

- sally quon

I am snow
heavy and dense
my weight crushes life
grinds worlds to a halt

I am snow
hard-packed and sharp
cold and unforgiving

I am snow
guided by the wind
seeking purpose
and a place to rest

I am snow
falling
I am falling

Am I the One Who Says I Am

Am I the I that says "I should"
the one who nightly cringes from regrets
the soaring spirit, the expanding mind
the fat, inert body
the tumbling mental chaos
deep breathing peace restored
gazing out at flowers, sun on water
childlike thrill of bird or beast
deer at the feeder
marmot by the road
magpie beeping his swoop across my lawn
this tangle of child, infant, adult,
crazy-turmoiled teen
depression, repression, anger, fear
unstoppable rage,
no matter how old I am
and still too old
and yet too young
so stupid so wise

Locksmith

by Dany Gagnon

I can't breathe
blood is locked in my throat
stopping the sounds I want to scream

I look for a key
to unlock the young girl
lost in the tricks of life

to extract my secret
a secret to restart my heart
to remember the wonder of being alive

The Stewing
By: Joshua Colenda

I stew,
On top of this fire,
With my ingredients inside,
Are they all necessary?

Some seem so bitter,
Some too hot,
Others dull.
My innards are painful,
Is this normal?

To stew on this fire,
With my emotions inside,
And pretend like I'm fine.
Who could enjoy consuming me?
When even I,
Do not like what's inside.

Am I to hang,
Here by myself,
With these poisons?

I look out over the kitchen.
So many empty pots.
How nice it must be,
To not have the fire,
Under your belly.
An empty pot,
Is all I want to be.
Lying on my side,
Cold,
And empty,
But happy.

I don't know what the point of every ingredient is,
But perhaps I can make the most of them.
Why would someone,
Include all these ingredients anyway?

Maybe if I change,
A this,
Or a that,
Or focus on the sweet,
Balancing the bitter.

Red meat,
And crispy onions,
Potatoes,
The ingredients I had forgotten,
Will balance each other,
And help me give strength,
To the people I love,
And make me,
A delicious meal,
For others to enjoy.

Biggest Fear

By Skye Ballantyne

Tell me your secrets,
Tell me your fears.
Tell me about the darkest parts of you,
That you don't share with anyone else.

I want to hear,
What keeps you up at night.
The sheet gripping fears,
That keep you up at night.

Maybe if I see your darkness,
I won't have to hide mine.
Maybe your darkness,
Can keep you from finding mine.

Maybe if I know the darkness
Inside of you,
You won't hate me,
You won't leave.

My biggest fear,
Is that you'll see me,
The way I see myself,
And you'll hate me too.

SOUL THERAPY

I cleanse the wounds with tears,
Erasing all memories of sorrow,
That buried deep within the soul.

I console the pain with verses,
Through lines of beautiful words,
In poems and tales full of meaning.

I calm the mind with adventures,
Venturing outside, observing the world,
Indulging myself for a moment.

I nurture the soul with prayers,
Seeking from the One above,
May the heart return to joy.

- **Lanzz**
Malaysia
22 November 2023

<u>When your eyes are infrared</u>
- Mark Heathcote

The Voices in Your Head
Say, I'm in control now, girl
just you, remember
when your eyes are infrared
you are with the devil wed.

You'll whirl with the wind
The fall leaves, turning red
You'll beat your poor head
Against some harbour wall
But there'll be no rest at all.

Every hour, I'll be moaning
Like some ungrateful lover
Who'll keep you chained, slaving
Over a hot, greasy cooker
Darling, every day will be Déjà vu.

You can throw such filth-
As excrement on the walls
But you can't eliminate me,
Remember, I hold all the keys.
Your illness is a disease.

And all those (DID) personalities
They'll have to remember not to squawk
Or talk bad-of-me
Or to the asylum house
In Bedlam, you will be.

Cheerless Morning

"Cheer", says the titmouse, "cheer, cheer"
so I try.
I cheer the sun, chill air,
the heavy morning frost,
try to find the cheer within myself.
It's not there.   empty   empty
hollow as a discarded bag
blowing in this wind.
If the wind can fill me,
why not the sun?
Why can't the cheer
reach deeper than my ears?

It is spring
and I am still winter's child,
rigid with ice,
empty as a torn plastic bag
fluttering in the wind.

Ever-Present (after Van Morison)

Bereft, place in society unsure
Dreamed that I died and no one gave a damn
And once again, this apathy murders
The ultimate opposite of true love
Missing the time I once felt acceptance
Belonging is anathema to me

And it's ever-present everywhere

Secluded, need to get away from home
It's dark and cold here, not enough layers
Stripped of my soul by lonesome hurricanes
Robbed my humanity with revolvers
Stared at the barrels, drank myself stupid
Illiterate, illumination ill
Screaming into the void, laryngitis
Voiceless, Darwinism is dominant

And it's ever-present everywhere

I navigate this city bulletproof
My words are durable like Kevlar vests
Enraged, engraved, epithets, ethics end
Alas, I'm all the more bitter and sad
Cried oceans, yet I heal and I survive
Warmth does exist even in these icecaps

And it's ever-present everywhere

Irreparable

by Carol Edwards

A little doll dangles
Limps from strings
The child I was changed,

In my calloused hands
A marionette stained –
Adult sins won't wash away.

"She's broken," I say,
"I cannot fix her."

Tears fall, break,

Water spots
In dingy carpet
Oceans of regret.

BOB

Bob opened the backdoor
of his Uber and wobbled off
toward the 24-hour CVS. His dress
was Dolce Gabbana. His heels were
Manolo Blahniks. He returned ten minutes later
carrying a bag of prescription estrogen; the trust fund
set up after all the hits he wrote in the 60's has kept him
well-fed, clothed and housed. He hung his head slightly
on his way back to the waiting car, and maybe it was
the reassurance of a successful trip to the pharmacy,
but the driver noticed Bob had the walk down
pretty well this time around.

Bob opened the car door,
slammed it behind him, let out
a heavy breath, loosened a heel and said:
"I just miss my late wife so much.
You have no idea."

Hate You

By Skye Ballantyne

I hate you
You made me feel
Worthless
Nothing I ever did
Was good enough.
I wasn't enough
Once
I was your favorite
Once,
I was enough
You made me feel
Like a failure.
You made me question
Who I was
You shattered
My self-esteem
And left me wondering
Why I wasn't enough

Self-Help Letter from a Friend
By: Joshua Colenda

My Friend,
I'm so sorry,
You are feeling,
This way,
But the answer,
Still is,
Hard work,
Every day.

With a reason why,
You can live,
Through any how.
It's awful you're in hell,
And I hope you make it out.

I'm here for you,
But I can't keep feeding you fish.
You need to be yourself,
If you ever want to live.
And I can tell you about,
Some things that worked for me.
But I can't lead you,
In fact,
I can barely see.

I want to help,
But I don't know how,
So here are some things,
I heard,
Wise men talk about:
If you fall off the horse,
Get back on,
Rome wasn't built in a day.
You reap what you sow,
So go plant some seeds.
Water them with sweat,
And then watch them grow.

I'm sorry you're in pain,
But please,
Don't end it all.
Someone out there,
Will buy what you can sell.
And if we lose touch,
I wish you luck,
I'll be here to talk,
When you get better.

Words
- Sally Quon

The words that know
even at dawn
which way the wind will turn.

Can you hear my voice?

breaking through the shadows
as a ripple of light
on still water

Do you see the moonglow
and behind it the fading stars?

hear the soft whisper of night,
inky blackness stretching on through eternity

I'm sorry.

Do you feel my hands
still holding the knife?

Where I'm Calling From

- Eran F. S. D. Hornick

About 16 menorahs
About 10,000 books
A brother
A mother born 40 years before me
A grandpa born 30 years before her
A taxi-driving, mainframe-programming, canoe-paddling father
A lake where loons call like specters on the placid water
That during gusts whips up to an angry roil
Reflections of blue moonlight on the watery ripples
A perpetually runny nose
A djembe whose reverberated noise damaged my left ear's hearing
Leaving me with a mild but manageable case of tinnitus
A book-recommending friend
A lego-building friend
A chips-and-tuna-eating friend
A friend we all turned against, ostracized, and banished, for what reason
    I barely remember
An Xbox, a GameCube, and a bunch of Pikmin
High scores in Tetris on Gameboy '92
My small rabbit with floppy ears
Countless flights to Florida, fanboats and alligators and a car that the
grandparents hardly ever drove
Walks to synagogue
220-mile drives to and from New York,
Brooklyn — Coney Island — being our destination
A collection of green-glass and clear-glass and amber-glass bottles
A homemade wooden box filled with world coinage
An album of stamps, then
2 albums of stamps
Then 3
A journal begun at age 5
Journal No. 2 at age 15
Then my sweet rabbit's untimely death

Trips to Canada: the Maritimes, Toronto, Montréal, the Laurentians,
Québec City.

Free printing at the high school library, thus no limit to my writing —
Hovering
Brooding over the printer
As the pages flew out, set in my favorite font, bleeding words from out
my heart.
Meeting Mr. Codish,
English teacher extraordinaire,
And his paper prompts on *Moby-Dick*:
"How to Render a Whale"
I scored an A++ on that one
Or were there 3 pluses?
Simpsons marathons with the Pipes
Shawshank and *Usual Suspects* and *Pulp Fiction* —
All the movies I'd missed as a kid —
At Martin's house on that double snow day in sophomore year.
Walking the eight-and-a-half miles home in the snowstorm with Alex,
when school should
definitely have been canceled.
Slaughterhouse-Five —
Hadn't known literature could do that.
My brother's multiple transfers through schools
Watching the 2004 Venus transit rise over Lake Michigan.
Senior trip to Israel, which took a turn for the brighter one day after a
particularly sumptuous
lunch.

Da Becks, playing his keyboard, my first friend at Brown
Wrestling on the ice
Hebrew lit and beginning Japanese
The tumultuous girlfriend and the ankle broken
Right before my flight to Japan
So I didn't go.
Frisbee
Monkey fist
And our first adventure — by hitchhike — to Newfoundland and

Labrador.

The job selling art, for nine-and-a-half years
The job saving turtles
For five
Traveling by thumb to Manitoba, to Idaho, to Northwest Territories and to Nicaragua
The fiasco of the Yukon
Weeks in Philly laughing with Ephraim
Girlfriends here and there
But none of them stayed.

Abandoning Boston
After bagging 24 summits in the Whites
After 12 visits to Douglas State Forest, mapping, ice-slipping, exploring with Shai
Driving Gwendolyn across Philly, Cincy, Chicago, and Great Falls
Pulling in to Albuquerque,
Exit 224,
And saying hello to teaching at Wingate
And goodbye to class of '22
And goodbye to class of '23
And hello to class of '24
And my folks' 42nd anniversary
Which I'll celebrate without them
At my friends' wedding, the same day, in Amsterdam Noord
Where I travel
On occasion
Though those occasions have become so frequent
That they spill over
From Journal No. 23
To No. 26,
No. 27,
Nos. 30 and 31
And the royal purple one, No. 32
And, soon, Escher's art-spattered one, number not yet assigned.

The beautiful, rambunctious niece

My dear Chana
The nephew
Bright little scamp Yehuda Leib
And the new niece
My angel Sima
And 12 flights in two years to go see them.

And age 36 around the corner – Year of the Rabbit again
And a flight tomorrow morning
To Amsterdam Schiphol
Where,
Surely,
They know me by name and by face by now.

Cocoa smoothies aplenty, with Lani, with Shai, with Laura
1,000 letters and postcards sent, received
In what I dubbed the Postcard Crusade
Begun in 2008
When we traveled to Yellowstone
And saw black bears,
Like that first time
Seeing the mom and two cubs dash
Across the road
In Shenandoah National Park, 1999,
In Virginia
Where Mom bought me some bear socks
To commemorate the date.

The Taste of You

- Dany Gagnon

Slowly the pixels fade away
leaving the city lights take over
through the half-closed blind
splintering on this oversized bed

the silence settles
as the anguish pours in
cold black ink
over my insides
    I want to resist
    I want to sink

spiraling down a tenebrous well
time trapped into a never-ending pain
the taste of metal in my mouth
I want to feel your final night

wrapping my heart
in this blanket of blackness
I am free from desire
to see beauty in desperation

yet enticing as it is I will come up for air
with the bullet still in my mouth
    to entwine my fretful mind
    lest it starts missing you

Waking Nightmare

By Skye Ballantyne

What happened
When you woke up?

A realization
Hit me

The realization
That I was awake

I didn't want
To be awake

I was having a much better time
Asleep

It was like a reverse nightmare
I woke up into a nightmare

- Tinamarie Cox

Bedtime Stories

Your words were bullets, coming at me fast, putting holes through me so I'd bleed the last traces of myself onto the floor at your feet.
Kneeling beside me with a smile, you tell me a convincing story of how you do it because you care too damn much, you just want what's best for me.
Playing nurse, you patch up the wounds you issued and fill me up with lies and fears and your toxic dreams, tell me a convincing story of who I am supposed to be.
You can only love the version of me I can't be without you, my careful puppeteer.

Grey moth

Grey moth, waiting its timely moment to fly
waiting its moment to swoon into a flame
takes to the air, while its life for a moment
is suspended in animation, hangs in deep despair.
It doesn't matter, it doesn't care, it hasn't a care
transfixed by some distant starlight's snare.

Only, it's not a distant star as it's now on fire
it's a vision of an all-consuming, transparent desire.
Grey moth, Grey moth, now it can't be found
I guess it has found in its-peculiar-way
what many today would fervently expound?

Call it madness or pure satanical-craziness
but there it has found sublime happiness
ah, contained it in its inimitable exultation
while headlong leaping into a fiery annihilation
Grey moth, Grey moth, now-it-can't be found
Grey moth, Grey moth, now-it-can't be turned around.

Learned to enjoy myself

by Henry Vinicio Valerio Madriz

Always… walking by myself.
Always… trusting my courage.
Always… following my own.
Always… learning about me.

Never… feeling lonely.
Never… getting desperate.
Never… hearing nonsenses.
Never… missing others.

Being alone but not lonely,
learning more about who I am,
thinking twice: my decisions,
loving the ways I am to
enjoy my own company,
it's just worth it!

The Island
By: Joshua Colenda

I am an island,
And I am barely around anymore.
I am sinking, starving.
My borders erode ever closer to my center,
And to nothingness.
Rivers and trees,
And all the things,
That make me unique,
Are being slowly being consumed,
By the waves.
Coming from without,
Reducing me to sand.
But suddenly,
My volcano explodes into action,
Sending my center,
Into the air all around,
It lands,
And hisses against the waves,
I am the one who makes waves now.
Soon,
The magma will cool,
And I will have more room,
To work with,
To be.
More for the world to see,
And my rivers to flow,
And my fruit to grow.
Until once again,
The waves begin consuming me,
Until my volcano rises,
And the waves,
Volcano,
Erupting,
Eroding,

Again,
And again.
The process is me.
And everything,
Against me,
And within me,
Against it.

Happiness Will Find You

By Skye Ballantyne

Everyone likes to say that
Happiness will find you,
When you least expect it.
One day you'll find happiness,
You'll realize that you're happy.
And that's probably true,
But what people don't say or don't realize,
Is that if happiness can find you,
So can everything else.
That means
That sadness can find you too.
Sadness finds you
Just as well.
It sneaks up on you,
Finding you in the darkness.
It finds you in your happiness,
And rips out the ground from underneath you.
Suddenly you find yourself
Falling through the air.
Your world begins to pass you by
In blurs of colors and sounds.
Nothing makes sense
As your life blurs together into meaningless nothing.
You are thrown into darkness
Not knowing which way is up.
You can't remember how it started.
You don't know when it will end.
You are turned upside down
And inside out
And left wondering
If you'll ever be able to
Stand up again,
If you'll ever find your footing.

Sadness if falling
Unstoppable
Never ending
It saps your life of meaning,
Takes away all the good things you've got.
Takes away everything,
Leaving you at rock bottom,
With nothing left
But to cry out for help,
and watch as people yell out,
"Save yourself."
They call out
Saying things about happiness and hope.
But they are all too busy
Going about their lives
Without realizing
It would be a lot quicker,
It would be more helpful
If they let down a rope,
If they lent a helping hand.
Yes,
Happiness can find you,
But you know what else can find you?
Sadness

ASYLUM

A Lady Macbeth
In disguise
Sleepwalking
Through dawns
And twilights,
Haunts the halls
And enshrouds
The withered
Frame
In insanity.
Now,
The shadows within
Struggle
To escape
The timeless body
Stiffened
By the walled
Doom.

Umbrellas

By Michele Rule

There's a line
where the wall meets the floor
that you mustn't cross.

Hold fast, dear one.
From the bright coloured world,
the images of your life
secured around you,
to nothing but

black and white.

Padded walls,
the definition of madness.

Yet there it sits
beckoning
on rainy days
in a whispered voice.
Just take an umbrella.

But once you begin
to explore that place
you can never come back.
I know,

just ask me.

Brightest Shade of Grey

- sally quon

Today I wore my brightest
shade of grey. Cold,
but not cold. Grasping
for a handhold on spider silk
hoping not to fall,

trying to outrun the storm.
Trying to outrun

thoughts, like salmon,
swim against the current,
spawn new generations, who ride
the water
back to the sea –

back and forth, back and forth.

Today, I am stretched thin,
jagged edges
tearing new holes
because the ones I had
weren't enough. Because
the scars I had
were beginning to fade.

Mice are Sensitive

by Carol Edwards

I live in constant fear the mice will come back.
The exterminator says they nest in the walls, but in summer they're off in the fields and vineyards.
He set traps for them.

I've had to clear and clean my cupboards ten times.
They rifle through closed canisters and bottles, like they're looking for something.
The most alarming was finding their traces in my closet, across shoes and under dresses, so close to where I sleep!
Do mice suffocate people? Eat them alive?
My stepmother complains I should just get a cat and be done with it.
She *doesn't remember* the terror she owned when I was young, how it attacked me, nearly taking an eye.
I still have the scars.

I live in constant fear the mice will come back.
The noises they make at night – scuttles and clicks and squeaks – roll like thunder to me, keep me from sleep.
My half-sister grouses I have rabbit ears, can hear conversations down the hall, made me difficult to play pranks on.
More like she tried so often it became a matter of course.
It didn't help stepmother took the lock off my door after Dad died.
"*Innocent fun*" is why I hate nighttime, have to take a pill despite the gate on my front door, the bars over my windows.

I live in constant fear the mice will come back.
I've had nightmares of mice for so long. Pumpkin-headed zombies crawl after me, hoards of brown and gray bodies pour from their eyes and mouths, vine hands reach to tangle my feet, and a limb heaviness pulls me down, every step a battle and so many steps yet to reach the chimney.
They hate fire, I somehow just know.

If I can light a fire and climb the chimney they'll disappear.

I live in constant fear the mice will come back.
So many times mice have ruined something for me: a birthday, a bus ride to town, a walk in the woods behind my house, even a trip to see my cheery godmother, Lord bless her, going a bit senile, still wearing glitter in her hair and waving her cane like a wand.
She says the mice are looking for Cinderella, probably panicked they're late.
She says, "You should tell them where Cinderella went; they'd be grateful. Mice and rabbits are awfully sensitive about these things, you know."
She likes to remind me of the time she found me feeding three mice off the back doorstep, crying as I chattered to them, pink dress muddy and torn, forbidden to leave the kitchen.
"You conversed with so many creatures then; what happened?"

I never told her the animals stopped talking back because animals *can't talk*.
I *made it up*.
I *overheard* things.
Stepmother gloats that she *broke me* of my *compulsive lying*, and how ever did my *poor father* manage, and see, wasn't she right when she *knew* I'd *ruin* Petunia's debutante Sweet Sixteen with a *tantrum*.
She wouldn't have met "*dear* Albert" and finally have the life she *deserves*.
"It was for the *best*," she says, "that Duchess killed all those mice in the attic. Cats bring carcasses of their kills to people they *love*, you know."

I live in constant fear the mice will come back.
That I'll find mangled bodies in traps, twisted corpses in corners that escaped the neck-breaking snap but not the poisoned cheese.
Why do they keep looking? They need to leave!
The ball is over, the glass shoes dashed, dress dumped in the trash.

Cinderella isn't here; she never was.

the border of us
- Michael Artemis

there's something here, lurking, hungry

there something out there, eating, teeth on show,
its eyes never closing, staring, licking your lips

there's something underneath us, sticking out from the ground, feeling the weight of the sun
on its shoulders while we sleep in flower beds, pulled down further
while we the two of us- four of us ate together on our backs, eyes never closing

there's something in the ocean, crawling on its belly, passing over crags that scratch
marks over skin, and it weeps in red, colours the gaps in, drags the sand out from underfoot
and doesn't let up, not for us, not when there's something behind us too,
we creatures of Innsmouth, we bread slicers, mundane watchers

there's something reaching out of us, hands creeping from mouths, forcing the bones aside,
much too large for us, clawing at blood-tears, the root
and you're two, the you dragged from you, smiling in red and teething,
the border drawn back, the remaining skin shucked off
and you are not you, lurking, hungry

Seasonal Affective Disorder (Sad)

- Mark Heathcote

So seasonal ills lull my every, mood
Ice flows inward outward my thinking
Never does the spring thaw lessen its rude
Hold on my life; each day begs, questioning.

How my overly anxious brain still ploughs on
Spirit frozen stiff and September
Four decays darker now just begun.
My emotions amplify the dread, December.

The 16th leading cause of death in females
Pulling at the fabric of my mind is Death
By suicide the eighth cause of death in males
The winter onset a stage for Macbeth!

Heartbreaker
By: Joshua Colenda

Although everything external's fine,
Everything's pessimist,
Here in my mind.
It's like,
Divine decree,
Saw all the things,
And said how things should be,
But,
I alone,
Misunderstood,
How hopeless things can seem!
Is it a factor of birth,
Am I on this earth,
To walk around lost,
And then die in the dirt?
So many people I see,
Roam around lost,
Come to a lock,
And then produce keys,
All except me,
Or that's what I thought.
But one day,
When the sun set,
I turned around,
In time to see,
An army,
Of opened doors,
Following me,
Like footsteps.
I ran around the planet,
In an attempt to understand it,
I talked to all the people,
Tried to figure who planned it.
And it turns out,

All the people that I talked to,
Everybody has the struggle,
That I struggle with.
And even those who made it through,
Know exactly,
What I'm going through.
But there isn't just a single way,
And so even,
If I listened,
As they gave me,
Their directions,
All our starting points,
Are different,
And our destinies,
Are different.
And though,
Nobody,
Can do it all,
For anybody else,
You can listen,
To how,
They made it through,
So you can help,
Yourself.
And then when someone,
Comes to you,
You can help,
Them too,
Because by then,
You won't,
Be selfish.
And one day,
When the sun rises,
You'll turn around,
In time to hear,
A crowd of strangers,
Lost,
Asking you for directions.

Peace

By Skye Ballantyne

I had peace.
I had hope.
Normal things,
People take for granted.

Slowly,
Those things
Began to slip away,
Leaving me trembling.

My world started caving,
Leaving me broken
Praying for an ending
To this never ending Hell.

Living inside of my head
The demons screaming loud
Telling me to let it burn
So I can find some peace.

The Popular Soul Who Feels Unloved

By Michelle Chermaine Ramos

You say you are friendless
and feel utterly unloved.
I see your heartbreak
unfolding in public posts
every time you beg for help to come
when you need it most.

That takes so much courage,
yet it pays off.

For then, your friends never fail
to come in droves
overflowing with love and encouragement.
My heart's inspired
as it both breaks and celebrates you,
for do you know how much
I admire and envy you?

For if my trembling voice
were to cry out right now,
with the same intense pain
and distress you bravely expressed,
I fear I'd only feel ashamed
if I'm met with deafening silence.

10:30

by: Natasha Alva

It was on a gloomy evening when you called me.
My heart was pounding in fear of what you're going to say.
I thought that my actions were silly jokes that can be played by.
Turns out, I crossed the line.
I'm glad you heard my story, but it wasn't enough.
Tried apologizing but being ignored for being bad made it worse.
Like a pest that can be swept away, it's a done deal.
With no messages received from you, I start to accept.
Since you and others saw me in another light, I'm banned from their existence.
It hurts when they only need you for something.
Despite receiving your forgiveness, the assurance of friendship is unclear.
I don't know if I'm able to trust myself in coming back to you.
Endless tears start pouring out, it won't make a fuss.
I will always be the outcast.
Good for you that there's a circle you can count on.
I'll leave you be as I have always been alone.

Addiction Diary: Entry 4: Detox

by Lisa Diaz Meyer

I live in addiction
So easy to swallow
No need to crush it
Or chew it
It just slides down
Straight up to my head
It closes my eyes
Even longer today
Who will care
If I sleep my lonely life away
And when I'm awake
I hate
And I hate
It wants me to despise
Conditioned me to despise
Until I taste the bitter bile
Of its mouth, not mine
It pours into my gut
My jaws grind an axe
The windows to the soul
They rattle
And they rattle
Everything hurts
It won't go away
You say I'm selfish
I say I'm in pain
Your meds play mind games
That changed the rules
I'll play your hateful game
I abhor how I need you

Impulse

- Michael Artemis

The impulse comes at 4PM when
you're passing a corner shop
with the vodka on sale.
Instead, you keep walking,
laugh like something stale
and dream. You buy
some bread and honey,
make your way home and
ignore the throbbing in your gut.
Next week you'll fall in love and hate yourself for it.
The corner shop shut down while you
blinked and the ash
is still in the gutter beside the door.
You gulp.
Love doesn't exist and you're lying in
the grass. A week later
on a dried up evening, the streetlights
smile at you. All you see is your breath in the air, and for a
second, you let yourself dream.
Pain is good, and
it's yours
to con
trol.

Villain Inside

By Skye Ballantyne

Every story has a villain. You have the wicked witch of the west, or the east, or the evil stepmother, or a monster, or a beast. There's always some villain, someone the hero must fight, kill, beat. My story is no different.

But who is this monster in my story? She's really hard to find. She's hard to see. She doesn't come with a big, black cape, or a witch's broom. There's no mask. No big sign telling you who she is. See, she's really good at disguises. In fact, she looks a lot like me.

"Mirror, mirror on the wall," I say as I look into the mirror, "Who's the fairest of them all?"

But is that quite right? I already know the answer. It certainly isn't me. It never is the villain of the story.

"Monster, monster, inside of me," I say instead, "Tell me, tell me, what you see."

That monster never fails me. It always answers my questions and makes me a prisoner. Traps me inside my own head as it rips me apart and tears me to shreds.

It brings out all my scars, all my pain, my sadness, my fears, and aggressions. It brings out all the horror I've caused and witnessed. It leaves me battered and bruised, leaving me with a void of nothingness that I can't fill. And makes me yell and scream into a silent void, taunting me with my own words, my own voice.

This villain isn't some mythical creature to fight or the devil sent from hell. It isn't a witch or a demon. It isn't some beast. It isn't something you can fight. It isn't something I can kill. But it's a villain all the same.

It's a villain that I can't defeat. It's a villain that will always win. After all, how do you kill the monster, when it lives inside of you?

Love is a Battlefield: A Dialogue

A Bottle of Gypsy Rose...His Story

Blew my mind,
On a bottle of Gypsy Rose,
And now I don't need no more,

Blew my mind,
On a six pack of brew
And now I don't need no more.

I'm thinkin' about givin' up,
I'm thinkin' about goin' straight,
I'm thinkin' about givin' up,
I'm thinking...maybe,
...it's too late,
...for me.

Blew my mind,
In a brown paper bag,
And now I don't need no more.

Blew my mind,
On some lazy grass,
And now I don't need no more.

I'm thinkin' about givin' up,
I'm thinkin' about goin' straight,
I'm thinkin' about givin' up,
I'm thinking...maybe,
...it's too late,
...for me.

Blew my mind,
In a white powder haze,
And now I don't need no more.

Blew my mind,
Ridin' that horse,
And now I don't need no more.

I blew my mind,
I blew my mind,
And now it ain't there,
...no more.

I Could Love You If You Live...Her Story

I could love you,
If you live.
But that doesn't seem to be.

I could love you,
I know it.
If only you could break free.

Lines down your arm,
Are doin' you harm,
They're killin' you and me.

I could love you,
If you live.
But that doesn't seem to be.

I could love you,
I know it.
If only you could break free.

It's fryin' your brain,
drivin' me insane.
And you're too blind to see.

I could love you,
If you live.
But that doesn't seem to be.

I could love you,
I know it.
If only you could break free.

Monkey got a hold,
Of your damn soul,
Chokin' at my heart too,
Hear my plea.

I don't think you see,
What our future could be,
But I'm not going down,
... all the way
...with you.

Static

By Michelle Chermaine Ramos

It's not baring my heart
in the depths of despair
that scares me.

It's the part where
I'm screaming,
and bleeding,
curled up in a ball,
bawling out my soul
into the world
pleading to be heard
and not hearing a single word.

Or even a faint echo
whispering back hello from a distant wall,
confirming that my desperate call
meant nothing to everyone after all.

Until you've suffered with it
- Mark Heathcote

When you've depression, abstinence
comes from not speaking, not eating,
not caring. But plenty of hard-drinking
when you've depression temperance-
is a lonely fictitious word out of verse.
No longer coupled with the meaning of this world
sobriety, isn't it just an oceanic bird
not yet drown, but in a self-denial
that it has been flying way too long?
Indulgence is a self-inflicted rushing tidal-
wave through the dense, thick fog, ere long.
No, it can't ever be confused with love.
When you've depression, there's no love-
can keep you safe above the waves that choke-
until you've suffered with it; depression is no joke.

DISORDER

By Olivia Arieti

When the will
Spins
In breath-taking
Whirls
With wistful
Eyes
You watch
Your other self
Fumbling
In the falling
Shadows
In search of
Lost memories
That melt
Faster than ice
And decompose
The mind.

Fireworks

When things are not preventable I try to be like water, scatter
                         back pinks and greens,
gold glitter, red like blood, shattered colors quiver to the sky.
It wasn't staged when I was a kid, only lightening or aurora,
                         rainbows, clouds, lots of those......
geese drawing lines, great clusters of blackbirds, snow, rain and stars -
 I've learned to reflect the long gold path the full moon paints.
Consider the Universe, or just the Milky Way -
we are very small.

The Day After

- Michael Artemis

When February 3rd comes around, Phil Connors, man of the hour, basks in his victory.
He's done it all. Gotten the girl, turned his attitude around, found peace in the mundane.
He orders an extra slice of pie for himself that day. Why not? There's all the reason in the world to celebrate.

When he enters the cafe, lovely Rita on his arm, the tinkling of the bell makes him

    pause.

Doris recognises the man who tipped her extra and gives him the largest slice they have.
This is perfect. He's figured it out. Rita shares a coffee with her perfect man. It's funny, he really did give her such an awful first impression.

She asks about his passions. About his dreams, the secret ones he has just for himself.
Once, he might have said money, deep pockets, a black card. But he is new Phil, the man evolved.
So he just shrugs, says he's working that part out.
Rita lets it go.

The second date is beautiful, a few miles out from the cherry street inn.
The conversation runs flat, but that's okay.
He's still new at this. It will take a while to sort out the little things.
After getting to repeat his trial run so many times, the awkwardness is fair trade.

A man he doesn't recognise
(he has to remind himself that new people are a part of life)
spills coffee on him.
Phil laughs, says he'll fix it next time.

    He stops.

His shirt is damp.
He will have to clean it tomorrow.

Phil has been silent for too long.
Rita is unnerved. She coughs.
Phil shakes his head. "It's nothing."
Rita doesn't buy it.

After a week, the dishes have piled up. Phil thought the morning would fix it.
Everyday, the pile gets bigger. Laundry becomes a daunting task.
His coffee stained shirt is flung to the ground, and there it remains.
Phil used to be good at living alone. Now Rita is being the Good Girlfriend.
Picking up the slack.
He can't bring himself to apologise. What good would it do?

Phil has a habit of saying the wrong thing.
When he stutters, he stops mid-sentence. Rita hates it.
The old Phil, for all his faults, never had a problem with expressing himself.
He was an open book of derision, but now he's pensive.
She's gotten jumpy in the night – Phil won't stop
shaking her awake.
"What day is it?"
His sweat is cold when he hugs her. It disgusts her. She hugs him anyway.

After a month of this, she unplugs the damn radio.
'I Got You, Babe' sends him into a panic. She's barely sleeping too, spends every morning
cradling him, rocking him, cleaning up his vomit.
Phil maintains that nothing is wrong. That he knows best, knows *Rita*.
And it's true – he knows things she's never said aloud, things kept between her and the pages of a diary.

She suspects him.
She fears Phil's temper, the panicked phone calls, the cloying hands at her night dress.
Rita misses the old Phil – craves their perfect day, Groundhog day.

In her grief, she turns to Larry. Sure, he's more Phil's friend than hers, but she needs someone like that. Someone who knows her Phil.
She's no cheater, and Larry's not her type – but when he puts a hand on her shoulder, she sags.
Smile dropped, tears falling.
Larry tells her she's not crazy. That Phil *is* different. No one knows what's wrong with the man.

She crashes on his couch.
A blanket has been tossed over her. Phil had never done that before.
He wasn't prone to consistent kindness, just grand gestures.

    Was that love?

She tossed it over in her mind.
It's been a year now. Has anything changed?
Was she doomed to live the same day, over and over?

When she goes home that night, the house is dark.
A single light shines from the bathroom.
Inside, Phil looks in the mirror, and hand on his head to pull back the hairline.
A single grey hair. He's transfixed by it. Unblinking.

Rita leans in the doorway. She thinks about how a little gray would suit him.
Her resolve is weakening.
"Want me to pluck it out?"

Phil doesn't turn to look at her. He doesn't even smile. "What would be the point? It'll be there tomorrow."

Rita purses her lips.

Tomorrow.

She'd like to go to the farmer's market tomorrow, pick out some cauliflower, some fresh herbs.
Once, she would have held her lover, invited him along. She knows better now.

"Have you been standing there all day?"
"I'll restart tomorrow."
"Phil-"
"You won't remember. It'll be okay."

Phil is quiet again. The tap drips.
Rita goes to the bedroom to grab her things.
She wants him to stop her. She knows he won't.

"I won't be here when you wake up."
Phil doesn't reply. Why should he?
He can try again.
He'll find a way to fix it tomorrow.
Tomorrow.
Tomorrow.

Demigod
By: Joshua Colenda

Worthless!
Alone in my room,
As depression surges.
What's the purpose,
of feeling the promise,
Of a better future?
It's a disservice.
The occasional glimpse of heaven,
Finds,
It's way,
To my conscious mind.
Never content,
It only suggests,
Teasing me,
Taunting me,
Tantalus.
Hope is a fire,
They brought to my psyche.
I pay for the price of that lie.
Everyday,
I stand on Olympus.
And look,
For the promise,
Delivered.
Eagles with talons,
And malice,
And beaks,
Come down,
To chow down,
On my liver.
One time,
They sent me to prison.
It wasn't my fault,
But they wouldn't listen.

It's just a condition,
They said,
Of cognition.
Of consciousness,
Knowledge,
Of language,
Ambition.
And just when I thought,
I had found my way out,
I took a look at the sun,
And then started to drown.
Never content,
It only suggests,
Teasing me,
Taunting me,
Tantalus.
Sometimes,
I feel like Atlas,
Holding the whole world,
Upon on my back.
Sometimes,
I feel like Odin,
Killing myself,
For knowledge potion.
Sometimes,
I feel like Sisyphus,
Breaking my back,
To get to the top,
Then watching my progress,
Roll down the hill,
And back to the start.
Never content,
It only suggests,
Teasing me,
Breaking my heart.
Maybe you feel like Medusa:
Beauty's a curse,
That leads to abuse.

Maybe you feel like Cassandra,
Who,
Always spoke truth,
But was never listened to.
Maybe you feel like Icarus,
With success so potent,
You're getting sick of it.
Maybe you feel like Atlas,
With the Earth on your back,
Filling you with madness.
Maybe you're a demigod too,
Half-god,
Half-savage.

Comforting You

By Skye Ballantyne

You're so quiet
You never say
What you're feeling inside
You don't talk
About the monsters
In your head.
You don't tell people
You're not okay.
Because it's hard
Watching them
Not knowing what to do.
In the end
You're the one
Doing the comforting
When the person
Who needs comforting
Is you

Unending

by Carol Edwards

I've forgotten how to exist
Caught between drops of rain
Or vapor mist rising
Where sound muffles itself into
A bass bubble
The thrum of my heartbeat
Out-shouted by the waves
Pressing me back together…

    Into pieces

        Vibrating apart at my atoms
        Losing molecules like
        Skin its own dead flakes
        Or pixies their dust
        Just strewn everywhere in
        Audacious glittering
        Though I don't think
        My little dark dots
        Could be mistaken
        For happy thoughts
        that make anyone fly…

            Though I might

            Into a rage
            Into the sky
            Away from the eternity
            That bumps into me at night
            Collides with my forehead
            Like I don't exist
            Not anymore

Trapped in this gray matter panic pattern
Over an un-ending.

"The Hundred Year War"
- Shevaun Cavanaugh Kastl

My life feels like the hundred year war.
Not everyone lived through it.
Spanning generations, intermittent invasions
Fought by endless variations
Of Me.
Serving time for subconscious naivety.
Disturbingly brief or insufferably long,
Like tragic but catchy old country songs.

Did this Me survive just to take a deep dive
Into past lives built for battle?
Perhaps that is why the most pained memories lie
In wait for future excavation...
For a Time to arrive when what's dead is revived,
Claiming strength of conviction and true benediction...
From graves buried deep like hangover sleep,
When my curious hand pricked the spindle.
Now I'm watching at the window.

I believe in my mind that I was designed
To endure my window pain.
It's easy to get lost when you live in rolling thought,
Slowly turning mad.
Am I good or am I bad?

Once upon a time, I was made out the villain
Red snow painted white.
Too good, too much, to make sense to You-
You who were always right.

My innocence curdled under your scrutinous stare.
You pilfered my hope chest until it was bare
And left me shell-shocked in an open cage,
Until all that remained was the echo of rage.

And a ghostly obsession with the line of succession
For a crown I never wanted.
Why then am I haunted?

What was it you said all those years ago?
Before terminal seasons of loneliness passed?
What didn't hurt then now pierces my heart
For fear that those words were my last.
No one will ever love you the way I do.

You left me pleading on my knees,
So smug as you uttered your cruel prophecy.
Would you be so kind Not to toy with my mind
That is reeling in feeling
And swallowed by meaning-

Did you know that I cry every night?
Scared to dare think I could lose this century's fight.

Shit.
I quit.

Paper treaties up in flames.
What was it We were fighting for?
That left me battered and sick to my core.
No matter, We lost it all in the end.
Switching roles like children playing pretend.
Victim, Victor, or Prisoner of War.
Always left for wanting more.

What hurts most is I fought for the right to my claim,
The one you renounced and called counterfeit pain.
You stood there above me, eyes red with vile
As I lay broken-hearted on blood-spattered tile.

But you were wrong.

I paid for my sins. I suffered my pain.
Not once, not twice, but again and again.
Not your paper cut penance
Nor stakes put to flame.
Contrition was watching my blood circle the drain.

Battle after battle.
To the torment of Death's rattle.

A War was fought. For a hundred years.
A War you thought you'd won.
But my ludic love you taught me this...
War is never done.

And so I soldier on...

Séance

    by Alex Grehy

I walk through the school canteen,
sliding my tray along like a planchette.

Is anybody there?

My identity, a translucent ghost,
cries out for acceptance.
The water in my glass shivers,
transparent, they look at me, through me.

The plump girls wearing glasses,
turn away; they think I've gone too far.

The pretty girls, the effortlessly thin,
scorn me with their pity,

The clever girls do not understand
my process.

The boys, who even now,
call me "fatty" to my face.

I tried to punch above my social weight,
by losing weight.

Diet, Gym, Run
Not Enough.

Starve, Binge, Vomit
Not Enough

Surgery, Infection, Scars
Not Enough

My bikini-flat body
not fit for a bikini

Never Enough.

They judge me unworthy,
who worked so hard to belong

I lie beneath them, a corpse of myself
lost in the soulless subsoil
between the beautiful and the mad.
Is there anybody there?
Does anyone care?

Because I am a Liar

by Carol Edwards

This thing I made for you
links a million little snowflakes
made of a billion folded planes,

Night holds them in her palm
so cold, diamonds with sharp edges
heavy and dangerous.

Day's touch undoes my work
the piles and layers I built
suddenly soft, tender,

a thousand x a thousand
showered from within
frozen Knowing rushes away,

Unknowing sinks to secret places
treasures, like snow, to grow
glow, wither – green lasts

only a little longer
serious earth and careless sky
loves and rivals.

This thing I made for you
frail with longing
trails the arc of my lying

across blue pages
light a herald of Life
and a gateway to ends,

unique in blindness, incapable

of describing the inside
of beauty – distorted shadows,

oil slicks, dissected birds' wings
one perfect flower undead in resin
a leashed star wearing lipstick.

This thing I made for you
glaciered maria
unsteady calves de-hinging

celestial bodies, or vice versa,
dissolves the moon: her glittering
tears unravel tides.

Originally published in Lit Shark Magazine Issue 5, June 2024

Are You Alive?

By Skye Ballantyne

I have launched myself from tall places
And hoped no one would catch me.
I have ended relationships
Because suddenly I felt too exposed,
And isolation felt safer.
Isolation would protect me,
But it didn't.
It's no safety.
It's a slow and painful death.
If no one knows you're sick,
If no one knows you're alive,
You aren't.

Dear old dead July

By Mark Heathcote

Dear old dead July, now it's August
you make me want to die
seasonal depressions they're here again,
they're here all over again.

Here, my weather vane
spins out of my control
my sundial has been turned over
year after year, now I no longer want to cry.

Dear old dead July, now it's August
you make me want to lie down and die
you make me want to weep, weep
like a willow longing to sleep.

My old house of golden corn
is now a shelled-out shell of an acorn.
The moon's darkness is bliss
I breathe it back into my lungs, a foggy, wet kiss.

Dear old dead July, now it's August
you make me want to die
curl, twirl crisp and crackle into the dust
oh, turn back time, turn back August.

Tightrope
    By Alex Grehy

He walks a tightrope
treading the wire by habit
strangely surefooted, gripping
the cord of his misery.
I see him close his eyes in anguish,
overwhelmed by depression
too stubborn to fall,
too frightened to change.

I stand helpless, feet on the ground.

I remember my fear
when he first stepped
on that taut wire,
remember reaching out
to pull him down, back.

But he refused my hand.

I thought of stepping onto
the wire behind him
but it was not the place for me.
I watched and pleaded
told him I would be his safety net.
He started throwing
objects down on my head -
spite, disdain, contempt,
heavy, hurtful.

Not all victims
of despair are nice.

I cried
ran away,

came back,
took the safety net,
the one that might
have saved him,
wrapped it round
my shoulders.

It's all that I can do.

Internal Monologue

by Carol Edwards

They read my text, I can see it
but they aren't writing back
   They usually write back.

        Did I annoy them?
        Do they not like me anymore?
        What if they don't like me anymore?!

                                    Hush; breathe.
                               They could be busy.
                                They work today.

But what if I annoyed them?
   Annoying is bad
dammit
I shouldn't have sent that last message
two was enough
I seem needy
   Needy is bad it's annoying
   Nobody likes needy
      I've lost another one
      Should've backed off
      let them text me
But they didn't seem
distant yesterday.

                        Something could have happened.
                              They're just busy.
                                 You get busy.

No, it's me
   It's always me
   I'm too much

    I'm too clingy why can't I be
    like everyone else?
        Why am I so desperate?
Oh god
they think I'm desperate
    Nobody likes desperate
        I lost another one
    How does this
        always happen?!
I'm hoveringbackoffflet them go
    It's okaythis is okay
        I don't carereallyIdon't
            This is good I don't mind it's fine
            It's better this way
        Just let goWhy haven't they texted yet?
What did I do wrong?
Am I toxic?
Am I the asshole?
It's not fineWhy do I always care so much?
    I care too much
    I'm so stupid
        Just let it go
        It's better this way
Yeah, it's better this way
  .
  .
  .

*ding

Self-Destruction

By Skye Ballantyne

The worst part
About anything self-destructive
Is that it's so intimate.
You become so close
To our addictions and illnesses.
They held us in our darkest moments.
They comforted us.
They were our shoulder to lean on
When no one else was there.
They calmed the voices
In our heads
And steadied the shakiness inside.
They were our confidante.
They helped us stand
While tearing us apart
They made us feel strong,
Made us feel empowered.
We were in charge.
They were our biggest support.
They became us,
So leaving them behind
Is like killing the part of yourself
That taught you how to survive,
And you don't know who you are
Without it.

Hide

    by carol edwards

There is a darkness
in the dips of light waves
and a heaviness
between the barbs of feathers
        (fake wings mistaken
           for things that can fly),

blindness tucks beneath
cones of red and blue and green
peeks out under moonlight's
softness, which makes us
not mind
        (like death lets
           the body not pay itself any mind),

and happiness glimmers somewhere
in the middle of a rainstorm
        (clouds livid and heavy
           eating and making mist)
droplets shining, the ribbon
on mountain peaks at sunrise:

        that's its game
                hide-and-seek

        (and it never really wants to be found).

Kind Eyes and the Loveliest Face I'd Ever Seen

by Gabriella Balcom

Two years old and scared to death, my heart trying to beat its way out of my chest.
My father's in the kitchen screaming! Now stomping down the hall, coming for me!
My room's tiny, the closet full. Nowhere to hide with his footsteps getting louder.
I crawl under my bed, scooting back as far as I can until I'm against the wall. I'd go
into it if I could. Mama's home, but I can't count on her anyway. She never helps me.
Never. I've seen dead animals before, and wonder if I'm about to die.

He's by my bed, still yelling. His feet mesmerize me. I struggle for breath, chest tight.
Surely he hears me. I cringe, waiting for the bed to be yanked up, but he walks away.
I stay hidden, lose track of time, but finally emerge. Silence surrounds me and I tiptoe
up the hall, stopping again and again, listening for the sound of his feet, his breathing,
anything. I discover my parents asleep in their room, but that doesn't change anything.
I don't feel safe. Never do. Hoping for a place he can't find me, I go outside.

His old car's parked nearby. It doesn't run and the darkness underneath beckons to me.
I crawl under the back, hear a sound, and freeze. Golden eyes are watching me. They're
warm, kind, and set in the loveliest face I'd ever seen. It's the tabby who's been coming

around. She's had babies and they squirm restlessly at her side. She hasn't moved yet,
and just studies me as I study her. When she mews quietly, I know she's talking to me.
I move closer and hear a faint, raspy purr. It's soothing and I drift off to sleep.

Life remains a living hell off and on, but there's a difference. I don't feel as utterly alone
and unloved as I did before. Day after day, I join Mama Kitty, and she lets me know how
happy she is to see me. I talk to her and she talks to me. She licks me and I pet her and the
furry little ones she trusts me with. I look forward to her company, read to her, tell stories,
and she understands. She was beautiful when I first saw her, but she's grown even lovelier
since then. Mama Kitty's the world to me, and she's my best friend.

The end.

Feel Alive

- Skye Ballantyne

The air is heavy.
Thick.
 I feel like I'm swimming through it.
Every movement is a struggle.
Every movement feels more energy than I can muster.
It's too exhausting,
 trying to wade through air this thick.

It's exhausting trying to breathe.
I often can't.
 The thick air chokes me,
 making it impossible for me to breathe.
My lungs ache as much as my heart does.

I feel so lost...so directionless.
 I don't know which way is up and which is down.
Don't know which direction
 I'm supposed to go.
I'm surrounded by darkness,
 without a light to guide me,
And no idea where I'm going.

My insides feel like they are being shredded,
torn to pieces,
tossed away
like a piece of trash.
And my soul.
 How do I describe my soul?
I can't.
All I can say is that it just...hurts.

Everything hurts.
My body hurts.
My soul hurts.
Breathing hurts.
 Living hurts.
I can't hold it in.
I can't take it.
 My tears stream down my face.
 I'm mentally grasping at proverbial straws,
 searching for anyone, anything,
 something that will help,
something that will ease the pain,
anything that will make this hurt less.

I know I'm grasping at straws,
 but please,
I just need something
Anything
to bring me to life.

IT'S NOT ME WHO WROTE THIS, ITS HIM, WE ALL HAVE DEMONS WITHIN.

by Aditya Pandey

It's my morning when the sun dies,
fireflies are my daylight,
I love it when the sky cries,
And the glowing tears in the moonlight.

I grin when the stars fall,
Looking at the empty sky in its dark form,
I hate the trees which stand tall,
Between me and myself, this damn wall,
My name calls.
and how I can't sit in a church's hall.

It's not me who wrote this,
It's him who made me do it,
It's him who, maybe, holds me,
Captive, In my own dreams,
Looks at me and says, now scream,
No one will hear you dying,
I say that he is lying,
Or maybe I just can't accept it,
My mind, I just can't reset it
I'm nothing but a prisoner,
Of myself, in my dreamworld.

Broken Glass

by Carol Edwards

Memories unbidden pester me
lurk behind corners
in the shadows of my daily routine
in shows I re-watch, places I've been.

They tuck themselves into folds
so thin
I forget they're there

the smallest thing a trigger
a sliver
splitting open
the snow globe moment
frozen in my mind
like I left a front door
gaping wide

nothing to keep secrets and shames
from pacing in
smearing footprints
over my finally-clean threshold
like they still own the place

their ghosts haunting habits
responses
coping mechanisms
trauma –
proof of what I'm trying to forget

what I'm trying to make submit.

I've spent so much time
sorting myself out, endless closets
of skeletons and boxes and precarious piles of junk...

Is there a point in trying to clear my head?
It'll just fill up again:

feelings with uneven edges
shaken until they shatter
jagged fragments
so small they burrow
lost
in gray matter cushion cracks
lying in wait
to bite tender unsuspecting skin.

Killing the Minotaur

- Dany Gagnon

Somnambulism and scribbling
same space same journey
do not wake me up
from either of them
breaking my lead
might get me to lose the thread
in my labyrinthine thoughts
and never wake up from the dream

Scared To Heal

By Skye Ballantyne

I'm scared.
Scared to heal.
Scared to move on.
To let my demons go.
They've been with me
For so long.
I don't know
Who I am
Without them.
They made me
Who I am.
They held me when I cried.
They were the only ones
That stayed
When everyone else
Disappeared.
They held me together,
As they pulled me apart.
They were the ones
That stayed.
I can't lose them.
Or I'll truly
Be alone.

about the authors

Shai Afsai

Shai Afsai is a poet and playwright living in Providence, Rhode Island. Enough said.

Natasha Alva

Natasha is a chemical engineering student who enjoys writing poems. Some of her poems are currently featured in the anthologies from Magkasintahan 2.0 Volume VII, Balm 2: Poetry for Beautifully Broken Souls, Forever September, Of Ink and Paper and Dream 2: Death, Despair and Happy Endings., Balloon Children, and Magkasintahan 3.0 Volume IX.

Olivia Arieti

Olivia Arieti lives in Italy with her family. Her poems appeared in Women In Judaism, The Wanderlust Review, Poetica Magazine, Eye On Life, VWA: Poems For Haiti, Cliterature, The Harsh And The Heart Anthology, Pagan Friends, The Expeditioner's Guide To The World, Bridging the Cultural Divide Anthology, Feile-Festa, Haiku Of The Dead, Obama-Mentum Anthology, The Ocean Waves Anthology, Red Penguin Books, The Seasons, Trouvaille Review, Poetica Clarendon House Books.

Michael Artemis

Michael Artemis is a horror short story writer and poet, currently residing in the North of England. Much of their writing inspiration for this collection comes from their lived experience with Borderline Personality Disorder. They have previously been published in another Red Penguin Collection - 'Dear You: Poems Through The Heart'.

Gabriella Balcom

Gabriella Balcom writes fantasy, horror, romance, sci-fi, literary fiction, and more. She's had 520+ works accepted and has five books out: On the Wings of Ideas (contract won after one of her stories was voted best in a book), Worth Waiting For (second place winner/2020 Open Contract Challenge), The Return, Free's Tale: No Home at Christmastime and Down with the Sickness and Other Chilling Tales. Gabriella's Facebook author page: https://m.facebook.com/GabriellaBalcom.lonestarauthor

Skye Ballantyne

I have always had stories in my head that needed to be released; stories that refused to be silent. They needed to be shared with the world.

Skye has a blog where she writes on a writing prompt each day. Check it out at:

https://scatteredthinker.weebly.com/blog

Joshua Colenda

Joshua Colenda is a sergeant in the US Army National Guard who lives in Salt Lake City with his two dogs. He enjoys hiking and playing guitar and has been writing and performing poetry since college. Colenda uses poetry as a vehicle to express himself and to talk about mental health issues.

Tinamarie Cox

Tinamarie Cox lives in an Arizona town with her husband, two children, and rescue felines. Her written and visual work has appeared in a number of publications both online and in print. She has two poetry chapbooks with Bottlecap Press, Self-Destruction in Small Doses (2023), and, A Collection of Morning Hours (2024). Her first full-length poetry collection, Through a Sea Laced with Midnight Hues, releases in 2025 with Nymeria Publishing. You can discover more of her work at tinamariethinkstoomuch.weebly.com.

Carol Edwards

Carol Edwards is a northern California native transplanted to southern Arizona. Her poetry has been published in myriad anthologies, print and online periodicals, and blogs, including Space & Time, Black Spot Books, Weird Little Worlds, Heart of Flesh Literary Journal, White Stag Publishing, and Lit Shark Magazine. Her debut poetry collection, The World Eats Love, released April 25, 2023 from The Ravens Quoth Press. Follow her on IG @practicallypoetical, Twitter/FB @practicallypoet, www.practicallypoetical.wordpress.com

Dany Gagnon

Dany Gagnon is a writer and translator living in Montréal. In the last six years, her poetry has appeared in over two dozen publications. She won Second Prize for the Polar Poetry Contest 2021, and also Second Place for the Mensa Canada Literary Awards (2023).

Alex Grehy

Alex Grehy (she/her) is inspired by a reflective life fuelled by her love of nature, rescue greyhounds, singing and chocolate. She is known for her vivid prose and thought-provoking poetry. Widely published, Alex hopes that her works will engage the reader's emotions and help them to make sense of the world around them. Her poetry collections, Last Species Standing and A Listener Speaks (Alien Buddha Press) are now available on Amazon.

Cherie Hanson

Cherie holds an MA in Contemporary American Poetry from UBC, Vancouver.
    Her non-fiction, Walking the Streets of Blood was accepted in 2019 for the Manuscript Intensive.

In 2021, she placed second in the Wine Country Writer's nonfiction Stan: Alone in the Attic.

In 2023, The League of Canadian Poets published "The Series" and Black Mountain Press published "Shattered Mirror", Her Story magazine.

In April 2024 two pieces were juried into "Red Eyes and Tired Lungs".

Mark Andrew Heathcote

Mark Andrew Heathcote is an adult learning difficulties support worker. He has poems published in journals, magazines, and anthologies online and in print. He resides in the UK and is from Manchester. Mark is the author of "In Perpetuity" and "Back on Earth," two books of poems published by Creative Talents Unleashed.

Eran F. S. D. Hornick

Originally from Boston, Eran Hornick has worked in sea turtle conservation, curating fine art, and weaving cane furniture. He enjoys puzzles and writing on his Royal Arrow typewriter. His published work centers on the natural world and the characters who navigate its rich waters and landscapes. He teaches college prep and literature to high schoolers in rural New Mexico.

Wanda W. Jerome

Wanda W. Jerome is an award-winning poet and author who channels spiritual messages in fixed and free poetry and prose during her morning meditations. Recipient of the 2024 Gold Medal from Military Writers Society of America for "Magical Morning Moments: Awakening to Love and Light" - a book of her poetry paired with gorgeous photography by Jasmine Tritten, an accomplished New Mexico author, artist, and photographer, Wanda calls the Sandia Mountains of New Mexico home.

Shevaun Cavanaugh Kastl

Shevaun Cavanaugh Kastl is a poet, playwright, and award-winning Actress and filmmaker hailing from Los Angeles. Her passion for storytelling, vivid imagination and dedication to developing her craft has earned the respect of both her literary peers and critics.

Lanzz

Lanzz is a new writer from Malaysia. His involvement in the writing world is just for fun, as well as a form of therapy. Prior to this, he has participated in more than 50 anthology book projects in all around the world.

Henry Vinicio Valerio Madriz

Born in Atenas, Costa Rica, 1969, Henry Vinicio Valerio Madriz is a teacher -English Teaching and Linguistics and Literature. Photography lover. He has published poems, short stories, and photographs, both online and print (in the USA, Canada, UK, India, Philippines, and Pakistan). https://www.facebook.com/henry.valerio.58/

Matt J. McGee

MATT McGEE writes short fiction in the Los Angeles area. His novel 'Hungry' is available on Amazon. When not typing he drives around in rented cars and plays goalie in local hockey leagues.

Lisa Diaz Meyer

New York writer, Lisa Diaz Meyer is the author of The All Roads Collection, an award-winning dark fiction short story and dark poetry series. Readers can also find her works in several anthologies published by Red Penguin Books, Local Gems Press, Bards Annual and Nassau County Voices In Verse. Visit lisadiazmeyer.com for more information, links and book availability.

Mary C. M. Phillips

Mary C. M. Phillips is a caffeinated writer and musician. Her work has been widely published in bestselling anthologies and journals. Two of her poems were selected in Lancaster Pennsylvania's Poetry-In-Transit campaign and can be viewed in Lancaster buses throughout 2024. Visit her at www.caffeineepiphanies.com.

Sally Quon

Sally Quon is a dirt-road diva, and teller of tales. Her work has appeared in numerous anthologies including "Better Left Standing," "Coming Out of Isolation," and Quills Canadian Poetry Magazine. Sally is an associate member of the League of Canadian Poets and a member of the Federation of BC Writers. Her first collection of poetry, Beauty, Born in Pain, was released in April 2023.

Michelle Chermaine Ramos

Michelle Chermaine Ramos (www.michellechermaine.com) is a multi-disciplinary artist, writer, and journalist based in Toronto, Canada. Raised in the U.A.E. and of Filipino, Spanish, and Japanese heritage, her poetry explores themes of cultural identity, spirituality, mental health, emotional healing, and self-empowerment. Through her art and words, she weaves narratives that reveal beauty and magic in everyday life.
 Instagram: @michellechermaine
 Facebook: http://www.facebook.com/MichelleChermaineArt/

Jessica Cook

Jessica Cook is a writer from Wiltshire with an MA in Creative Writing. She lives with schizoaffective disorder.

Kit Rose

Kit Rose has been writing since she could hold a pencil and will be writing until she can no longer work her hands. Creating and helping others make their creations come to life is the embodiment of who she is, and she is eager to share that with the world.

William John Rostron

Born and raised in Queens, NY, William John Rostron now splits his time between his home on Long Island and traveling the country in his Tiffin motorhome. He is busy completing a bucket list of travel adventures when not writing. In the past 20 years, he and his wife, Marilyn, have traveled 140,000 miles. These journeys have taken them to the 48 contiguous states, 133 national parks, all 30 major league baseball stadiums, 154 cities and towns, two Canadian provinces, and various unusual experiences and locations. Many of these locations have served as backgrounds for his books.

He is presently working on a fifth novel, Dancing with the Lost, which may be read independently or as the fifth book in the Band in the Wind series.

www.WilliamJohnRostron.com

Janet Rudolph

I have written several books including When Moses Was a Shaman, When Eve Was a Goddess, and my autobiography, Desperately Seeking Persephone. I write wherever and whenever I can to express, heal, inform, challenge, startle and to expand love. I am a contributor and co-weaver at /feminismandreligion.com/ My latest project is She Speaks: Women of the Bible Have Their Say.

Michele Rule

Michele Rule is a disabled writer from Kelowna BC. She is especially interested in the topic of chronic illness. Michele is recently published in Five Minute Lit, Spillwords, Poetry Pause (LCP), and Chicken Soup for the Soul, among others. She is an associate member of the League of Canadian Poets. Michele lives in a beautiful garden surrounded by people who love her. Read more of Michele's work at www.linktr.ee/MicheleRule

Jaki Sawyer

I have always loved poetry and have written for many years. Born in Alberta, I lived in various small towns for the first 39 years of my life, then married and moved to New Hampshire for the next 26. Retired and moved to Kelowna in 2014. I have been published in several anthologies and magazines.

Deepika Singh

Deepika Singh is from Margherita Assam India, qualification- Master of Arts, B.Ed and teacher by profession. Her writings reflect her personal observations of day to day life. She believes that the right words can change our society. Her work got published in various national and international publications and some of her poems were translated into Spanish, Chinese and Serbian language etc. She also recited poems in BBC radio Kent.

also from the red penguin collection

Fiction

What Lies Beyond – Sci-Fi Stories of the Future
I Can't Find My Flashlight – Contemporary Campfire Stories
A Heart Full of Love – A Collection of Romantic Short Stories
Behind Closed Doors – A Mystery Anthology
Once Upon A Time… – A Fairy Tale Anthology
Ernest Lived …and other Historical Fiction Short Stories
Until Dawn – A Supernatural Anthology
Treat-or-Trick – Halloween Horror Stories
Pets On the Prowl – An Animal Mystery Anthology
My Robot & Me – A Not-So Fiction Anthology

Poetry

'Tis The Seasons – Poems to Lift Your Holiday Spirits
the flower shop on the corner – A Spring Poetry Anthology
the ocean waves – A Summer Poetry Anthology
the leaves fall – An Autumnal Poetry Anthology
Proud to Be – A Pride Poetry Collection
Words for the Earth – A Poetry Project
Dear You – Poems Through the Heart

The Stand Out Series

Stand Out – The Best of The Red Penguin Collection, Vol. 1
Stand Out – The Best of The Red Penguin Collection, Vol. 2

www.ingramcontent.com/pod-product-compliance
Lightning Source LLC
Chambersburg PA
CBHW060601080526
44585CB00013B/650